Help, We're Pregnant!

The Ultimate Guide to Preparing for your Baby

Introduction

I want to thank you and congratulate you for downloading the book, ""Help, We're Pregnant!: The Ultimate Guide to Preparing for your Baby."

This book contains proven steps and strategies on how to be prepared for each month of your pregnancy.

The 12 chapters in this book contain important information on what you can do to keep yourself and your baby healthy and safe throughout the 9 months. Learn the proper diet for a pregnant woman, how to prepare for your prenatal visits, the types of safe exercises that will help make labor and delivery go smoothly, and so much more. Let this book be your guide all the way from the first month up to labor and delivery.

Thanks again for downloading this book, I hope you enjoy it!

Chapter 1 – The Primary Steps during Pregnancy

Congratulations! At this point you must have already confirmed that you are pregnant. You might have taken a urine or blood test, a medical exam or a home pregnancy test and it came out positive.

Well, there is absolutely no need to fret. Having a baby is a very normal part of life. Beautiful and healthy babies are being delivered every single day, right this very second in many hospitals and homes around the world. This book will guide you throughout your journey of pregnancy, from the first month up to the labor and delivery day. Assuming that you picked up this book shortly after knowing that you are pregnant, we shall thus start at the very beginning.

Take a Vitamin Pill, ASAP

The very first thing that you need to do now that you are pregnant is to take a prenatal vitamin pill that has folic acid, calcium and iron. To be more specific, look for a prenatal vitamin pill that contains the following:

- Maximum of 4,000 IU (or 800 ug) of vitamin A

- Minimum of 400 to 600 ug of folic acid (folate)

- 250 mg of calcium

- 30 mg of iron

- 50 to 80 mg of Vitamin C

- 25 mg of zinc

- 2 mg of copper

- 2 mg of vitamin B6

- Maximum of 500 ug of vitamin D

- Approximately 15 mg of vitamin E, 1.4 mg of thiamin, 1.4 mg of riboflavin, 18 mg of niacin, and 2.6 mg of vitamin B12

Make Lifestyle Changes

Also, you can already start making changes in your lifestyle for the benefit of your baby. These include:

- Setting a reminder to take your prenatal vitamins regularly

- Not drinking alcohol

- Not smoking

- Avoiding areas with secondhand smoking

- Stop drinking more than two cups of coffee and herbal tea regularly.

- Stopping any highly restrictive diets

- Getting at least 8 hours of sleep

Set your First Doctor's Appointment

Another important thing to do as soon as you found out that you are pregnant is to call and schedule your first doctor's appointment. Keep in mind that the busier a doctor's clinic is, the farther your scheduled appointment will be. Sometimes, they will set your first prenatal visit on your 6th week of pregnancy.

However, if you suspect that you have a high-risk pregnancy (based on your medical history), inform your doctor's clinic so that they can squeeze you in for an earlier appointment.

Know your Health Care Professional

If you have not decided yet on who will be the one to help you deliver your baby, the first thing that you can do is to determine what kind of patient you are. To do that, try answering the following questions:

- Are you willing to put all your trust on your doctor in making decisions (sometimes even without consulting you)?

- Do you want all of the best medical technology to be used in your care?

- Do you believe that you should ultimately be in charge of your body and health?

- Do you prefer minimal interference from the health care professional?

If you are more inclined to respond yes to the first two questions, then you might prefer the more traditional practice wherein it is the doctor makes the decisions. If it was the latter two, then you would want a practitioner, certified nurse-midwife or direct-entry midwives who will work hand-in-hand with you throughout the process. If you are at a dilemma towards all four of these questions then you can opt for a professional who is a good balance between the two different qualities.

Choosing the Type of Practice

Once you have decided on the kind of health care professional that you want to work with, the next step is to choose the type of medical practice. There are five different types for you to choose from.

Solo medical practice. The doctor is independent, which means that you will be seeing the same doctor in every visit and be able to build a good relationship with him/her. The problem would be if he/she is not available, a new practitioner might be the one to deliver your baby; another would be if you end up not liking your doctor.

Partnership or Group Medical Practice. At least two doctors work together in providing you with care, which increases your chances of knowing the practitioner who will be delivering your baby in case the other one is not available. The problem would be possible different points of view from different doctors. Another is if you don't like any of them.

Combination Practice. One or more physicians along with one or more nurse-midwives compose this practice. The pros and cons are similar to that of the partnership or group medical practice.

Maternity center-based practice. The physician is on call while the nurse-midwives do most of the work. Only low-risk patients are admitted in this type of practice. It is a great option for those who prefer primary practitioners or certified midwives. However, the problem would be if there is a complication during the pregnancy and you might need to go to a different physician altogether. Also, if there is a complication during your delivery then you will have to be transported to the emergency room of a nearby hospital.

Independent certified nurse-midwife practice. If you have a low-risk pregnancy you can avail of an individualized prenatal care and a natural delivery. Nevertheless, it is imperative that the independent CNM has an accompanying physician who will be available for consultation in the event of any emergency.

Have you decided on the type of medical care for your pregnancy? Do not be afraid to ask questions and do extensive research before you make your choice. Ask friends and relatives who have recently given birth and medical care professionals that you know personally for their advice.

Chapter 2 – Eating for Two: The Pregnant Woman's Diet

A pregnant woman's diet is one of the biggest factors that will contribute to the health of the baby. Of course, a nutritious food is the way to go. The great thing about following a healthy diet plan is that it will help increase your chances of a comfortable and safe pregnancy and postpartum recovery as well.

Important Dietary Tips for Pregnant Women

Commit yourself to a healthier diet by making simple changes in your meal choices. Here are some tips on what to do and where to begin:

Be conscious of all that you eat and drink. Everything you put into your body will affect your growing baby as well. Before considering certain foods that you know are unhealthy for you and your baby, think of better alternatives instead. For instance, you can opt for whole wheat instead of white bread, fat-free frozen yogurt instead of ice cream, kale or soy crisps instead of potato chips and grilled instead of fried chicken.

Eat five to six small meals a day. Spacing your mealtimes and minimizing your portions will give you and your baby a steady supply of nutrients without making you feel bloated, constipated or heart-burned. Try this: divide your breakfast, lunch and dinner meals into two and eat the divided portions between 2 to 3 hour intervals. That would give you a 1st and 2nd small breakfast (6AM and 9AM), a 1st and second small lunch (12NN and 3PM), and a 1st and 2nd small dinner (6PM and 8PM). Or you can have small breakfast, lunch and dinner meals then have 3 small, healthy snacks in between.

Choose healthy calories. There is more than just calories that you should take into consideration when it comes to choosing foods; the amount of nutrients in those calories is just as, if not more, important. Avoid empty calories (foods that barely have any nutrients) because these will only make you gain weight but not nourish you and your baby.

Absolutely no crash diets. As long as you eat healthy, you should not worry about getting fat. You can worry about dieting and exercise after you have given birth. Also, it's perfectly alright to give in to a slice of chocolate cake every now and then as long as you prioritize nutritious meals 9 times out of 10.

Daily Nutrition throughout your Pregnancy

Your baby will need only around 300 calories a day, which does not necessarily mean that you double up on your helpings. This makes it even more important for you to choose nutritious foods in order to make those 3oo calories really count.

To start off proper nutrition throughout your pregnancy, here is an overview of all the servings that you will need and why:

Protein- 3 servings a day (total of 75 grams). The amino acids and other nutrients in protein are essential for your baby to grow healthy and strong. Keep in mind that protein is not limited to meat alone; whole grains, legumes, nuts, seeds and dairy also contain high amounts of it.

Calcium: 4 servings a day (total of 1,200 mg). Calcium is a necessary nutrient for the development of your unborn baby's bones, muscles, heart and nerves. It is also required in blood clotting and enzyme activity. Not getting enough calcium will make your body draw it out of your own bones to help facilitate your baby's growth.

Vitamin C: 3 servings a day. This very essential vitamin is needed to help repair tissues, heal wounds and enable your body to perform other metabolic processes. Your baby will need it for the development of bones and teeth. Since Vitamin C cannot be stored by the body, you need to have a constant supply regularly.

Whole grains and legumes: at least six servings a day. Whole grains are full of the B vitamins that are essential to your baby's growth. Complex carbohydrates also contain iron, zinc, magnesium, selenium and other trace minerals that you and your baby need every day.

Leafy green and yellow vegetables and fruits: four servings a day. From these foods you will be getting beta-carotene, which plays a critical role in cell growth, leading to healthy skin, eyes and bones. Aside from that, you will also get trace minerals, calcium, vitamin E and a host of B vitamins, including folic acid and riboflavin, from these vegetables.

The rest of the fruits and vegetables: two servings a day. Fruits and vegetables that do not fall under the leafy green and yellow category are still chock full of magnesium, potassium and other trace minerals that you will need throughout your pregnancy. The rule of thumb is to pick a rainbow of colors for your plate; the brighter the color, the more nutritious it is.

Iron: 30 to 50 milligrams or 60 to 120 milligrams (for anemic women) a day. Iron is needed for the formation of blood, which you very much need as your body continues to provide for your developing baby. Combine vitamin C with iron as the former helps your body to absorb the latter more efficiently.

(Saturated) Fats: three to four servings a day. Your pregnant body needs essential fatty acids that will help your body absorb the essential nutrients from the other foods. But be careful not to overdo it as you can already get your steady supply of fats by adding a tablespoon of vegetable oils, butter, mayonnaise, creams or peanut butter to your plate.

Fluids: at least 64 ounces a day. Our bodies, including your baby's, is made up mostly of fluid. It helps keep us moisturized, eliminate toxins and waste products, and distribute nutrients throughout our bodies. Aim to drink water frequently throughout the day, along with some fruit and vegetable juices as well as milk.

Chapter 3 – The First Month

The first 4 weeks is usually a time when you still feel like your usual self, apart from the pregnancy symptoms that have already started to come out, such as breast tenderness and nausea. At this point, some women do not even know that they are pregnant! Nevertheless, the first month is a great time to go to your first prenatal visit, telling your family, friends, co-workers and/or employers, as well as making some changes in your lifestyle.

Your First Prenatal Visit

The first time that you meet with your health care professional for your pregnancy will be quite a long visit. You will be going through some procedures that will help you prepare for the development of the little one that is growing inside.

The first thing that your practitioner will do is to confirm your pregnancy and your estimated due date. You are also going to be taking another pregnancy test.

Second, he/she will interview you a great deal to notate your complete medical and history, including allergies, chronic illnesses and previous surgeries. You will also be asked about your family medical history, personal gynecological history, obstetrical history, and so on. Your practitioner will also inquire about your lifestyle habits so that he/she can recommend the necessary changes.

A complete physical examination will be the next step, starting with a general check-up of your heart, lungs, breasts and abdomen. Your blood pressure will be recorded along with height and weight. Signs of varicose veins and edema will also be inspected. Next, the doctor will check your external genitalia, vagina and cervix by using a speculum, as well as your pelvic organs. This will help him/her assess how the delivery will go based on the conditions and measurements.

Do not hesitate to raise questions regarding your health and pregnancy. Your practitioner will be happy to address all of them in order to help ease any concerns that you might have.

Routine Tests for Pregnant Women

There are common tests that you might be required by your practitioner to go through, while the rest are up to you. Here is a list of the tests related to your pregnancy:

- Blood test in order to determine whether you have anemia or not, as well as your blood type, Rh status and HCG levels.

- Urinalysis to check for protein, white blood cells, blood, bacteria and glucose

- Blood screens for determining the anti-body titer or levels as well as immunity to certain diseases such as rubella

- Pap smear to check for signs of cervical cancer.

- Blood sugar level test to determine risk of developing gestational diabetes or for existing diabetes.

- Tests to check for signs of infections, including HIV, syphilis, hepatitis B, gonorrhea and Chlamydia.

- Genetic tests for genetic diseases such as cystic fibrosis, Tay-Sachs or sickle-cell anemia.

Your Baby's Development

Within the first month, your baby should look like a little tadpole that is all curled up and as big as a grain of rice. The head and a mouth opening will already be present, as well as a heart and a rudimentary brain. The arms and legs will only be tiny buds.

Chapter 4 – The Second Month

The period between 5 and 8 weeks is usually the time when many women actually begin to suspect that they are pregnant since they have missed their period. If you are already aware at this point then you might still be trying to get used to the new lifestyle that comes with the pregnancy.

Start to become more cautious with what you eat, and always sanitize thoroughly before and after meals. Never eat any meat, fish or eggs that are not being refrigerated and if you are cooking, you must always wear rubber gloves to avoid cutting yourself and getting an infection.

Avoid eating anything that is raw, not even runny scrambled eggs. Wash raw fruits and vegetables thoroughly and avoid eating sprouts as these are usually contaminated.

Your Second Prenatal Visit

In order to prepare for your baby and make sure that your pregnancy will go smoothly, it is highly advised that you visit your doctor at least once a month. Make sure to write down the symptoms that you have been feeling beforehand because your doctor will want you to talk about these.

A second exam is likely to take place during your second visit, although it will be a much shorter one compared to your first. Your doctor will most likely take the following tests to check up on your current state: weight and blood pressure and your urine to check for glucose and protein. He/she will also examine your hands, legs and feet for signs of edema and varicose veins.

Possible Symptoms during the Second Month

Not all women experience the same symptoms. In fact, most women do not experience any symptoms at all. However, the feeling of being pregnant would usually kick in during this period so going through the following symptoms is completely normal.

Many women find themselves feeling the need to urinate more frequently and even experience constipation. Nausea, exhaustion and sleepiness are felt more often than usual. Headaches will also be experienced on occasion. Breasts become heavier, fuller and the areola will begin to darken. You will also notice that the veins in the breasts to become more prominent.

Bloating, flatulence, heartburn and indigestion are also common symptoms. Your food cravings will start to come in, as well as aversions to certain foods that you used to eat without a problem.

Your baby bump still won't stick out at this point, but you will begin to feel that your clothes are too tight, particularly around the waist area.

Your Baby's Development

Your uterus will be the size of a grapefruit by now, and your little baby will be about an inch in length. The embryo will also resemble the form of a baby this time, not a tadpole anymore. The little tail is gone, and the fingers and toes would start to stick out at the end of the 8th week. The eyes are now there, although the eyelids are still shut, as well as the ears, the tip of the nose and the tongue. The major organs and systems are now formed, but not completely developed. The baby has already started to move in reflex.

Chapter 5 – The Third Month

You are now at the final month of your first trimester at approximately 9 to 13 weeks. Any symptoms that you might have felt in the previous months might still stick around at this point.

However, the great news is that those pesky feelings of nausea would usually go away at the end of this month. Even greater news is that you will finally be able to listen to your baby's heartbeat in your next prenatal visit!

The Third Prenatal Visit

Make sure to have a list of questions ready for your doctor before the visit. He/She will be doing his/her usual check-up to see how your body is coping with the changes, such as measuring your weight and blood pressure and have you take a urine test to check for glucose and protein.

You and your partner will also get a chance to listen to your baby's heartbeat for the first time. The size of your uterus will be measured via external palpitation in order to check whether it is in line with your due date. The height of the top of the uterus called the "fundus" will also be examined. Finally, your arms, feet and legs will be checked for signs of inflammation or varicose veins.

Weight Gain

One of the most significant factors during this stage is the weight gain. By the end of the 13th week, you will have a weight increase of around 3 to 4 pounds. It will then gradually increase at about 1 pound every week. However, it is also normal to notice that you are gaining half a pound in one week and then 1.5 pounds in the next. Keeping track of your weight gain will help keep you from over- or under eating. However, if you notice anything unusual related to your weight even if you have been following a healthy diet, make sure to inform your doctor.

Your Baby's Development

From approximately 9 to 13 weeks, your baby will transition from being an embryo to being a fetus. You will be able to feel your waist sticking out already since your uterus would be a size larger than a grapefruit.

The baby would be around 2.5 to 3 inches in height and 1.5 ounces in weight by the 13th week, and about as big as an apple. The neck will have already been formed, which means that the baby's head is no longer attached in between the shoulders. The hair pattern has begun to form as well. The eyes move closer to each other and the ears start to become prominent. Tiny, soft nails have begun to form on the fingers and toes, as well as taste buds in the tongue. The sucking reflex, along with the sex of your baby, will also be present.

Chapter 6 – The Fourth Month

The fourth month is officially the start of your second trimester and it is often regarded as the best trimester by many pregnant women due to many reasons. First, most of the early pregnancy symptoms will be disappearing. Second, you become more accustomed to the new lifestyle. Third, and probably the most exciting of all, you will start to get a real baby bump.

The Fourth Prenatal Visit

Your doctor will be doing the regular checkups that were enumerated in the third month. However, make sure to have a list of unusual symptoms that you have been experiencing, along with early pregnancy symptoms that are still present.

Notice that you will no longer be getting headaches; only fatigue will come to you at times. Your urge to urinate would become less frequent, however, as well as the "morning sickness" that comes with nausea. Some women might still be experiencing constipation at this point.

Working Out while Obviously Pregnant

Exercise should still be very much a part of your daily life even if your belly is already protruding. Ask your doctor about the different exercises that he/she would recommend. Exercise is very important as it would not only keep you from becoming overweight during the pregnancy but also help ensure a successful delivery, especially if you are aiming for a natural birth as opposed to a C-section. However, if you are in a high-risk pregnancy you will most likely need to avoid strenuous exercise. Again, talk to your doctor before attempting anything.

Some exercises that are proven to be safe for most pregnant women are the following: brisk walking, swimming in shallow water with room temperature, simple water exercises, Pregnancy Yoga, Kegel exercises, relaxation techniques, and stationary bike cycling using light or moderate tension and speed.

If you feel that you do not have enough time for exercise, a simple 20 to 30 minute walk in the early morning or early evening (to avoid the blazing hot sun) with your partner will do you good.

Your Baby's Development

Your baby will be about 5 inches in height and 5 ounces in weight. The body's growth will begin to catch up with the head and become a bit more proportionate. The fingers and toes will be quite distinct, and the lanugo (which is your baby's temporary hair) will have grown all over the body. The baby might also start thumb sucking, swallowing amniotic fluid, and do reflexive breathing. Your baby's bones will become stronger and the arms and legs will already start to move around. Soon enough, you will feel a kick!

You would be able to feel your belly protruding at 1 and a half inches below your belly button by the 17th week since the uterus will be as big as a small melon. Naturally, this would mean a change of wardrobe for you.

The placenta will be fully developed and functional, providing nutrients and oxygen to your baby. If you have a baby girl, her ovaries and primitive egg cells are forming.

Chapter 7 – The Fifth Month

Any time between 18 to 22 weeks, you will start to feel your baby moving around and probably even kick. Your belly will be quite prominent by now as well, making you feel very much pregnant. Apart from the fetal movement, you will begin to notice a significant amount of white-colored vaginal discharge called "leukorrhea", and it is completely normal.

Your Fifth Prenatal Visit

Your check-up will not be so different from the one that you went through last month, although it is always best to make a list of symptoms so that you can inquire about them to your doctor.

Inform him/her about the leukorrhea, any nosebleeds or ear stuffiness that you might have felt, leg cramps and possible bleeding gums. You might also notice that your heart rate has increased and varicose veins might have started to appear on your legs. Some women also experience developing hemorrhoids at this point. Although these are considered to be common you should still inform your doctor.

Getting an Ultrasound

Many practitioners would recommend, or even order, a pregnant patient to undergo an ultrasound. This can become a routine process that needs to be done once every 20 to 22 weeks in order to gain reassurance that everything is perfectly alright. Do not worry about whether the ultrasound will harm your baby or not, for it is guaranteed to be risk-free and will harm neither the fetus nor your pregnant state. However, it is advised that you consult your doctor before you go to store-front ultrasound studios since some technicians might not have undergone formal training and might even misinform you about the state of your pregnancy and your baby's.

Your Baby's Development

Around the 20th week, your uterus will be large enough to touch the back part of your belly button. The baby inside will be from 7 to 9 inches in length and would weigh almost one pound. The bones continue to grow stronger and the nerve system starts to develop, which means that your baby will be doing movements more frequently (even somersaults!). Your baby's ears will already be prominent and are capable of hearing. Even sleep and wakefulness are already being experienced within the womb. The skin of your baby will be covered with "vernix", a slippery white substance that protects your baby from the amniotic fluid and will make delivery go more smoothly. If you are having a baby boy, his testicles will already be descending from the abdominal cavity.

Chapter 8 – The Sixth Month

At about 23 to 27 weeks old, your baby is big enough for you to feel his or her movements quite significantly. Light exercise should only be the ideal fitness routine as your body continues to change in order to adapt to your growing bundle of joy.

You are probably going to start feeling some aches around the lower abdomen as well as the sides due to the stretching of your ligaments in order to accommodate the uterus. Your ankles and feet might start to swell, and sometimes even your face and hands. Your navel will be protruding at this point if not earlier on, and your skin will start to pigment around the face and abdominal area.

The Sixth Month Prenatal Visit

This will be similar to the previous months, with the routine check-up of your blood pressure, weight, urine, and uterus. Your baby's heartbeat will also be checked. By now, you might have already developed the habit of writing down any concerns that you might want to ask to your doctor.

Preparing for Childbirth

It is highly recommended that you and your partner attend a childbirth class in order to be educated in accurate information regarding normal labor and delivery, as well as the likelihood of complications, medical procedures and interventions, and so on. The sixth month would be a good time to start attending this type of class. Most childbirth classes also include relaxation techniques, muscle control and breathing exercises to prepare you for labor and delivery.

A childbirth class will enable you to bond with your partner as well as other expectant couples who can share their thoughts and stories with you. This is also a great time for you to bond with your partner and to let him understand this incredible experience that you are going through. This would help him become more involved as well as orient him on what to do and how to feel throughout the process of labor and delivery.

Most women learn to become more confident after attending childbirth classes because they are educated on how to handle the stress that often comes with labor. This can be quite empowering and the self-esteem and relief that comes with it will benefit both you and your unborn baby.

Your Baby's Development

Your baby will be approximately 12 inches in length now and a little less than 2 pounds. Walking and pedaling reflexes would kick in, as well as the gripping reflex; some babies even grip the umbilical cord, but don't worry for this is perfectly alright. The eyelids can open and close and the eyes have become more sensitive to light. The vocal chords are fully functional; although there won't be any sounds coming out until the baby comes out.

Chapter 9 – The Seventh Month

This marks the onset of the final trimester, and it can be quite an exhilarating time since there will be lots of preparing to do. Check-ups during your prenatal visit will be the same as usual except for a possible Glucose screening test and blood test to check for signs of anemia.

Glucose Screening Test

At around 28 weeks, it is usually part of the routine for doctors to recommend a glucose screening test in order to check for signs of gestational diabetes. There is no need to fast for this test.

You will need to drink a sweet glucose drink an hour before they take a sample of your blood. If the results come out showing signs that you have gestational diabetes, it means that your body is not producing sufficient insulin to handle the excess glucose in your system. This will lead to another test, called the glucose tolerance test, wherein you will need to fast and then drink a stronger dose of the glucose drink before another sample is drawn.

Around 4 to 7 percent of pregnant women have gestational diabetes, so if you have been careful with your diet and exercise then the odds are in your favor.

Creating a Birthing Plan

A birthing plan is a list of what you and your partner are expecting from the hospital or birthing center during labor and delivery. This includes the following specifications: locale of your labor and delivery, whether you can go out of bed, eat and drink during labor, having a personalized atmosphere during labor, presence of a camera or video camera, delivery positions, c-section, use of forceps or vacuum extractor, immediately holding and breastfeeding the baby after delivery, and so on.

After creating your birthing plan, discuss the details with your doctor so that if there are any necessary changes in the future you will understand that it is for the benefit of both you and your baby.

Your Baby's Development

Your baby will be gaining weight quickly from here on. In approximately the 31st week your baby will be 3 pounds and 16 inches in length. The lanugo will be fading away and will only be present in the back and shoulder areas. Hair will start to grow along with eyebrows and eyelashes. The lungs are also starting to function.

Chapter 10 – The Eighth Month

This is the perfect month to enjoy your pregnancy for the weeks ahead will be quite busy as the due date draws near. Bond with your partner and family as often as you can since all your (and even their) attention will be focused on the new baby once it is born.

Routine check-up will be performed during your prenatal visit except for the highly recommended Group B strep test.

Group B Strep Test

Group B strep infection is caused by a bacterium that is present in the vagina. Carriers of this infection will not be harmed. But a newborn baby might be infected as it passes through the vagina during natural childbirth, and this can be dangerous.

There are no symptoms of the infection and only a test can determine if a woman is a carrier. Even if your doctor does not recommend it, it is advised that you request for it.

The test is conducted the same way as the Pap smear using both a vaginal and rectal swab. If results come out positive, you will be given IV antibiotics as you go into labor. If the infection is found in your urine, you will be given prescription oral antibiotics.

Your Baby's Development

Your baby is from 18 to 29 inches long and weighs approximately 5 to 6 pounds. He will continue to gain half an ounce per day. He will look very much like the baby that will be coming out soon, with wrists, neck, and dimples fully formed. Since he or she is quite big now, a lot of kicking and wriggling will be felt. Your baby will also be experiencing REM sleep and active wakefulness as the brain continues to develop at a fast rate.

Chapter 11 – The Ninth Month

It is the final month and you must be quite excited and nervous at the same time. You probably even have a pile of baby stuff in the new nursery that you and your partner have prepared so carefully for the new addition to your family.

The last prenatal visit will be another routine check-up as before, but be sure to have questions prepared especially regarding Braxton-Hicks contractions. Your doctor will be giving you the delivery protocol as well, and if he/she doesn't make sure to request for that.

Packing your Hospital Bag

Here is a list of all the things that you will want to pack up in a nice, sturdy bag and bring to the hospital or birthing center:

- A compilation of notes on standard procedures and medical information of you and your baby.

- Copies of your birthing plan for attendants.

- A list of phone numbers.

- A timer for timing contractions.

- A camera or video recorder if you want to capture the moments.

- A plastic rolling pin for your partner to use for massaging you in case of backaches.

- A laptop or tablet for movies and games to entertain yourself (or any other form of light entertainment).

- Toiletries: toothbrush, toothpaste, mouthwash.

- Comfortable, nonskid slippers and heavy socks.

- A comb and a hair band to keep your hair in place.

- Nightgowns or robes that you won't mind getting stained.

- Maxi pads (never use tampons)

- Several pieces of underwear and nursing bras.

- A supply of healthy, easy to eat snacks.

- Extra set of clothes for your partner or guardian.

- Your clothes for going out of the hospital.

- Baby's clothes for going out of the hospital: a kimono, booties, receiving or bunting blanket, and diapers.

- Infant car seat.

Your Baby's Development

In the final two weeks before your due date, your baby's size and weight will already be considered as "full term" or ready for birth. Weight will continue to increase from 2 to 2.5 pounds and body fat will have a 15 percent increase. Most likely, your baby will move into a head-down birthing position. If not, ask your doctor for advice on how to encourage this. Sometimes, regular light walks for 20 minutes will let gravity help your baby into this position.

Chapter 12 – Labor and Delivery

After nine wonderful, albeit challenging sometimes, months you are finally about to give birth to your little one (or more than one). Naturally, this is the most anticipated moment for both the mother and the father.

So many concerns are probably swimming through your mind, especially regarding when the labor will start and when it will end. This chapter will guide you through the stages and phases of labor so that you will become more aware of what will happen and put your mind at ease.

The Stages and Phases of Labor

There are three stages of labor, and the first stage has three phases:

Stage 1: Labor

Phase 1: Latent or Early. This is the longest phase, but rest assured the least painful one. The opening of the cervix is around 3 cm and the thinning out (referred to as "effacement") that signifies this phase can span from days to weeks. Contractions are not even apparent, and if they are they are not overbearing. These contractions generally last from 30 to 45 seconds. As the due date becomes closer, the contractions gradually increase as well. Make sure to time your contractions, starting with the beginning one the first and then the beginning of the next one for 30 minutes if they seem to be about 10 minutes apart.

You will experience backache and you might have diarrhea a blood-tinged mucous-like discharge. It is possible for the amniotic fluid to rupture before the contractions start.

At this point, it is best to stay relaxed and make yourself comfortable throughout this process. Observe how you feel and do not call your doctor until you are in active labor, unless you are otherwise advised. You should also contact your doctor directly and immediately if you notice any greenish discharge from the amniotic fluid, bright red blood, ruptured membrane or absence of fetal activity.

Avoid eating too much during these times, and choose only the foods which are easy to digest such as broth, fruit and toast.

Before the onset of active labor, make sure to plan a route from your home, workplace or any other place you frequent during this period. It is sometimes better to call a taxi when the time comes for you to go to the hospital as parking can be difficult. Make sure that you and your partner or guardians are oriented on the standard admission procedures of the hospital or birthing center beforehand as well.

The moment you are close to the end of the early phase (with contractions at approximately 5 minutes apart), you will need to get to the hospital or birthing center. Have your partner or guardian constantly stay in touch with you around these times for you should never try to go to the hospital on your own.

Phase 2: Active Labor. The second phase typically lasts from 2 to 3.5 hours, although anything longer or shorter may still be considered normal. Contractions will be much more intense, longer (at approximately 40 to 60 seconds) and successively (at 3 to 4 minute intervals without a significant pattern). It is important to be in the hospital or birthing center by now.

You can begin performing the breathing exercises that you have learned, unless they do not make you feel at ease, in which case you do not have to do them. You can drink water or suck on some crushed ice if you feel parched, but only if your doctor allows you to. If you are hungry, you can ask your doctor if you can have some jell-o or applesauce.

Do not hold back your urge to urinate; it is imperative to relieve yourself as soon as possible. You can walk around and shift positions that make you feel the most comfortable. Do your best to remain calm for you will need to reserve your energy for the delivery.

Phase 3: Transitional Labor. Contractions will become even more intense during this phase. They will come in strong waves between 2 and 3 minute intervals and from 60 to 90 seconds long. Dilation will expand from 3 cm to 10 cm gradually from 15 to 60 minutes.

There will be intense pressure in the lower back and perineum area. There will also be pressure in the rectum, a sensation that feels like an extremely intense urge to move your bowels. Legs will become cold, trembling and prone to cramps. Drowsiness will set in, accompanied by nausea and possibly vomiting. There might be a tight sensation in the throat and chest area.

Remember to be very brave at this point and to remind yourself that millions of women successfully overcame this phase. Soon enough, your baby will be born. Be careful not to push if you are not instructed to do so; what you can do instead is to pant and blow. Pushing before full dilation will inflame the cervix and delay the delivery.

Stage 2: Delivery of the infant

Pushing your baby out is a natural process caused by the reflexes of your cervix and uterus. Listen carefully to your doctor and be guided by his/her careful instructions. Do your best to push because the more you put yourself into it, the faster the delivery will be. Focus your energy on the area below your belly button and envision yourself exerting effort from there. Maintain a relaxed upper body to avoid chest pain. Do not feel embarrassed because all women who go through natural labor went through the same process. All the pain and hard work will be worth it once your newborn baby is brought to your arms.

Stage 3: Afterbirth/Delivery of the placenta

Pain is gone, your beautiful bundle of joy is out and all that is left is for the placenta to be pushed out by your body. It can take from 5 to 30 minutes and you will barely feel it. You will naturally feel tired from the labor, but an overwhelming sense of relief as well. At this point, you would not even care except to cherish this moment and bond with your baby.

Cesarean Section

There will be times when c-section is necessary. Sometimes you would already be anticipating it, but other women who are initially expecting to have a natural birth would have to turn to c-section if complications arise. However, trust that it will be a safe and smooth process. If it is an emergency c-section, expect everyone to be moving about in a much faster pace. Try to remain calm throughout.

Your abdomen will be shaved and sanitized before the operation. Sterile drapes will be curtained around your abdomen so that you do not have to see anything. IV infusion will follow, as well as anesthesia, which can either be an epidural or a spinal block.

Once the anesthesia is in full effect, incisions will be made. The baby will then be eased out carefully by hand or using forceps. The cord will be clamped and cut.

The doctor will check on your reproductive organs and then stitch up the incisions. You might be injected with oxytocin afterward to help the uterus contract and lessen the bleeding. Standard hospital procedures would then follow.

Conclusion

Thank you again for downloading this book!

I hope this book was able to help you to prepare yourself for the wonderful months ahead. Pregnancy is an amazing part of a woman's life and giving birth to a healthy little baby (or babies) is even better.

The next step is to continue to take care of yourself and seek professional guidance so that your practitioner and/or birth class coach can help tailor-fit their advice to you and your baby's needs.

Finally, if you enjoyed this book, then I'd like to ask you for a favor, would you be kind enough to leave a review for this book on Amazon? It'd be greatly appreciated!

Thank you and good luck!